Welcome

TBI HOPE MAGAZINE

Serving All Impacted by Brain Injury

March 2017

Publisher
David A. Grant

Editor
Sarah Grant

Contributing Writers
Tobie-Lynn Andrade
Nancy Bauser
Nick Dennen
Molly Dorhauer
Ralph Poland
Mandi Seipel
Mike Strand

Amazing Cartoonist
Patrick Brigham

*FREE subscriptions at
www.TBIHopeMagazine.com*

Welcome to the March 2017 issue of TBI HOPE Magazine!

We are moving through another national Brain Injury Awareness Month. This month marks our seventh as a survivor family. I say "survivor family" because no one recovers from a brain injury alone.

What better month to share some news about something very exciting happening here at The TBI HOPE Network?

Starting next month, we will be offering a print version of TBI HOPE Magazine. We will always offer the digital version of our publication for free, however many readers have asked about a printed version of the magazine a reasonable cost.

You asked, we listened!

Readers will find the same hope-filled content they've come to love, in a full-color magazine format. I'll be sharing more details soon!

We are currently looking for regular contributors from the medical/professional community. If you would like to share your knowledge with the brain injury community, we'd love to hear from you. You can email me personally at david@tbihopeandinspiration.com if you are interested.

Though Brain Injury Awareness Month is winding down, you have the power to advocate all year. Your story has value and I encourage you to share it with others. You never know whose life you may affect for the better!

David A. Grant
Publisher

Contents

Supporting the Brain Injury Community Since 2015

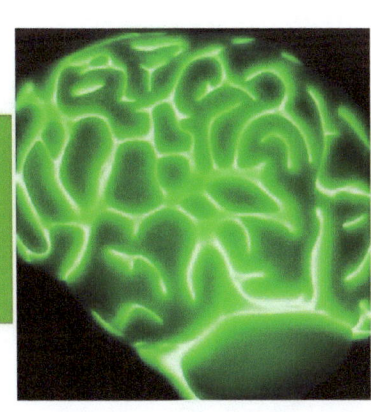

Healing with Harry Potter

By Tobie-Lynn Andrade

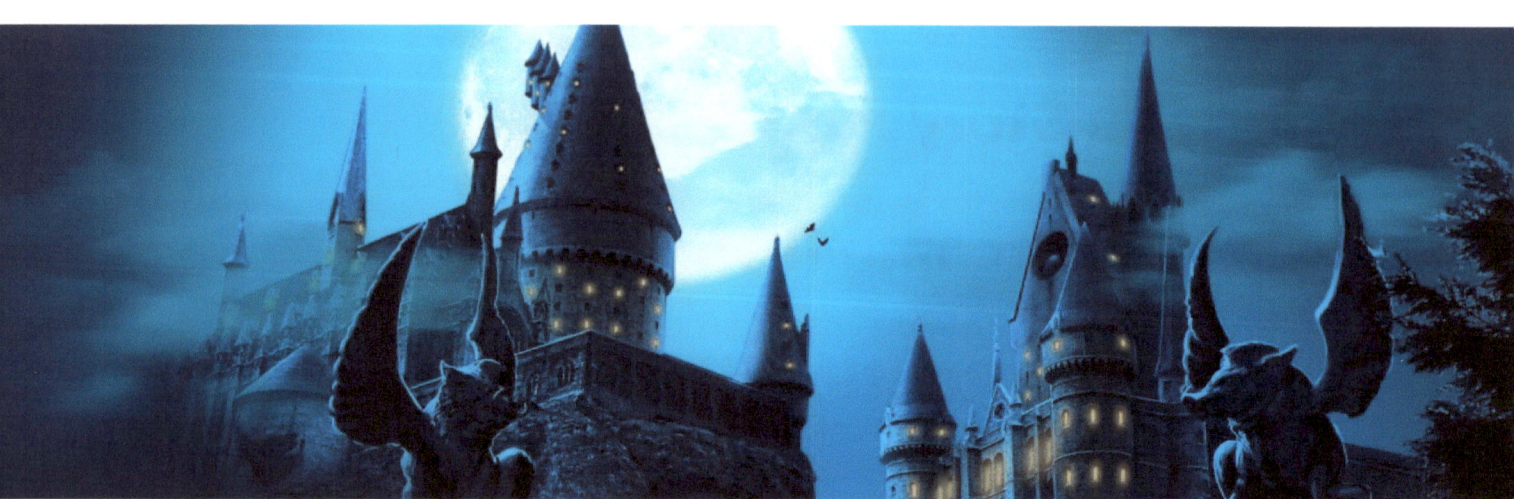

I have always enjoyed the wizarding world of Harry Potter, love my memories of reading the books with my sons, going to the theatre as each of the movies came out, and watching and re-watching them at home. My husband and I even spent our honeymoon at the Universal Studios theme park in Orlando, so we could visit the Harry Potter attraction. I didn't realize how something I enjoyed, something that brought relaxation and comfort, would help me heal after my head injury.

All injuries are different, as are all healing cycles. I had difficulty with language – reading, speaking and comprehending. As someone with a lifelong love of books, I was devastated to be searching for words, stuttering, and not understanding what I had just read. I was so fortunate to have been given the advice to start language therapy with something I knew – for some, it's lyrics or psalms – for me, it was Harry Potter.

I was so familiar with the words of the books, it felt like coming home – it was peaceful to read them again – so what if I couldn't regurgitate each thing as it happened – I knew the story and could follow the book even if I couldn't remember a page or chapter. I was able to read again and not feel frustrated; it was safe and fun. It made me feel good to complete a book.

I used it to speak again. I read the books aloud to my pets, to my husband or just to myself. Speaking the words was also oddly freeing – I knew them, and even when I would stutter or slur I felt comfortable enough with the content to continue. It raised my confidence. I started to speak more clearly. I had less trouble when I had to read lists aloud, and eventually talking aloud became less of a struggle as well.

It could have felt weird or immature or silly, but it felt like I was doing something.

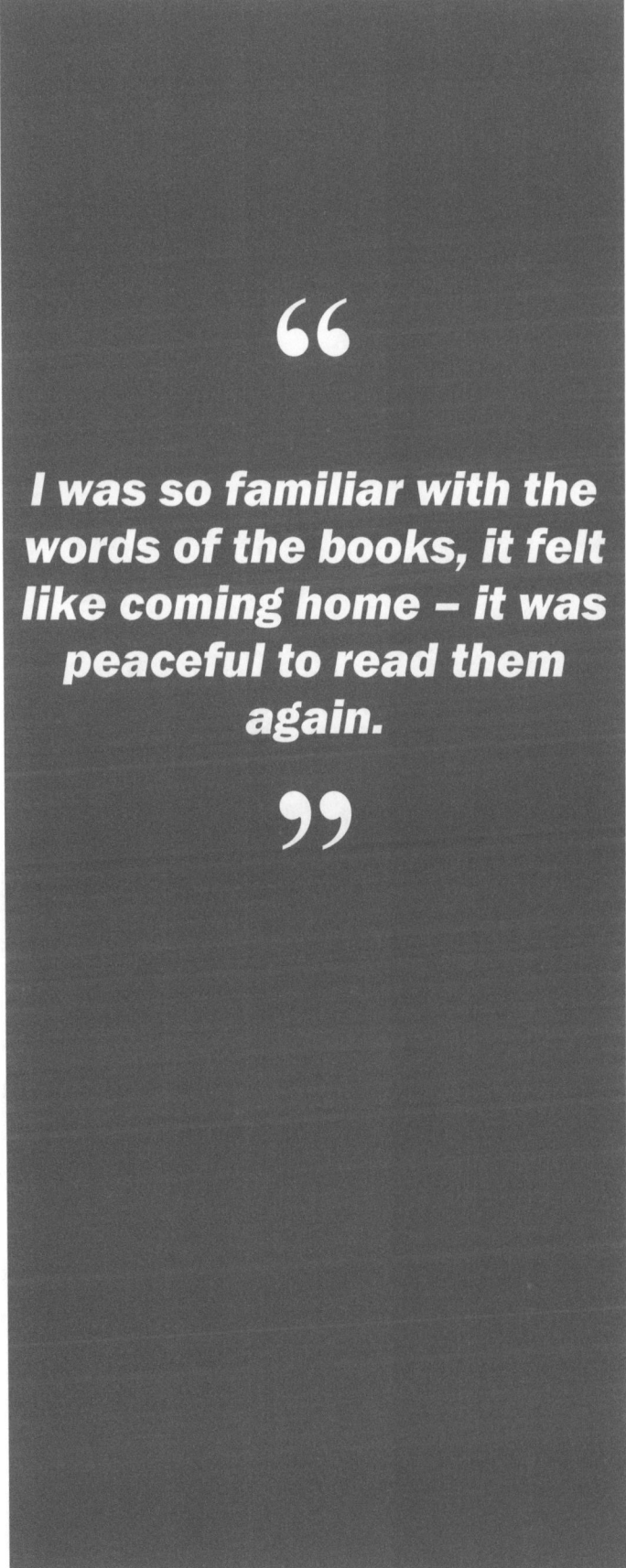

I was so familiar with the words of the books, it felt like coming home – it was peaceful to read them again.

I knew these stories, the characters, and the words and since it was comfortable it worked.

I used it in other areas of my recovery too. Always an avid crafter, I found myself struggling with instructions. Physical dexterity and the complexity of laying out fabric according to patterns was overwhelming. I couldn't visualize what I was supposed to do.

My same helpful therapist suggested Lego's. Yes, the building blocks. I scoffed at first, but my supportive family got on board and got me some (you guessed it) Harry Potter Lego kits. I actually struggled a lot at the start but was able to use the images in the instructions and my inner child took over.

> *"Reading, comprehension and spatial reasoning were just a couple of ways I used Harry Potter inspired healing."*

Suddenly I was physically building something and it made me feel strangely successful and fun. Anyone who's recovered from any kind of injury knows "fun" is not usually part of the equation.

I was able to take the relearning of the visual to the physical building process and use it in my daily life in ways I didn't think were related. From Lego's, I progressed to sewing patterns, other craft activities and even assembling some IKEA furniture.

Reading, comprehension and spatial reasoning were just a couple of ways I used Harry Potter inspired healing. For myself, I get very quickly and easily overwhelmed with noise and visual stimuli. It was difficult to watch even short clips of the movies or to hear the audio books, but I was gradually able to increase my tolerance.

It's always easier to pause a movie you've seen and come back to it than it is to stop something new and pick it up again. Plus, knowing the stories helped

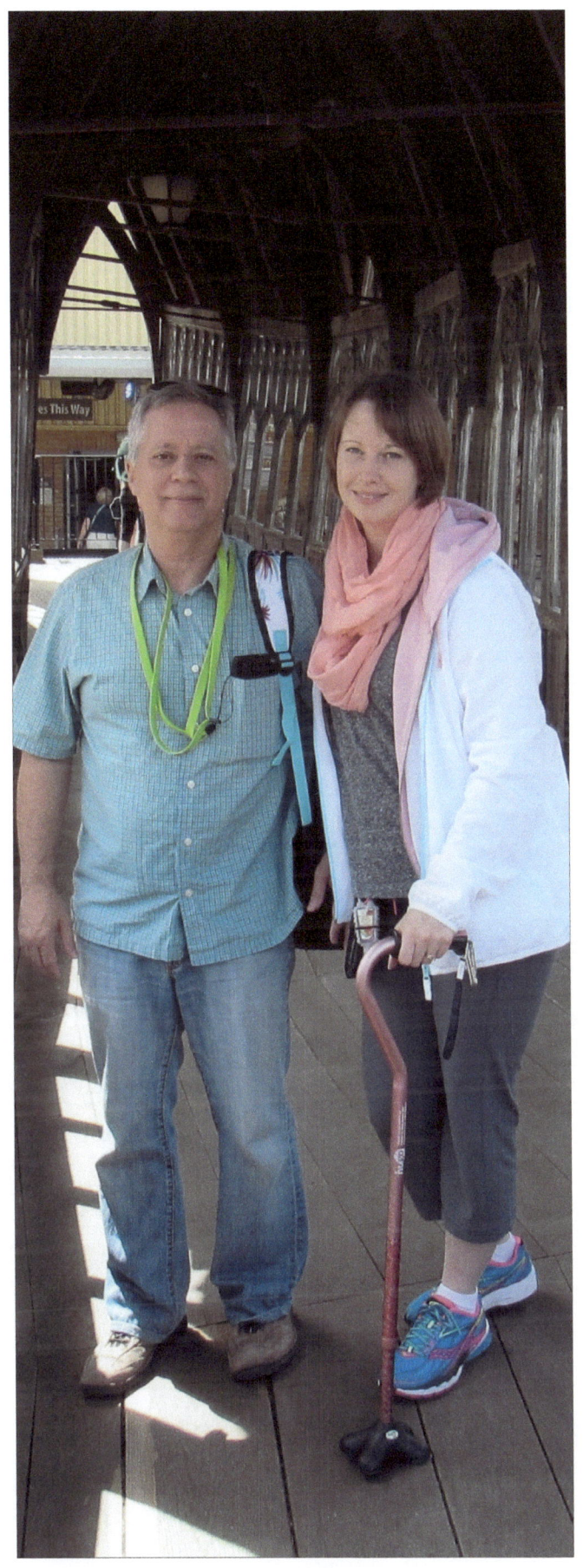

me to catch up again and understand what was going on in the rest of the movie.

Physically, my challenges came mainly in the form of seizures and walking disturbances. After a particularly brutal episode of such seizures, I was paralyzed from the waist down, hospitalized, and came home in a wheelchair. I worked hard to graduate to using a walker, eventually a cane. My family offered unconditional support throughout that phase of my recovery as well and they gifted myself and my husband a vacation to celebrate my being able to walk again.

It was a bucket list dream of mine to see the studios in England where the Harry Potter movies were filmed, and once I was able to walk with a cane my husband and I enjoyed the trip of a lifetime to make my dream come true.

I still use the Harry Potter stories in my recovery daily. I am at a point now where I am trying to increase my multi-tasking skills; listening to an audio book while sewing or having the movie on in the background while knitting. Even new learning is coming more naturally now.

I love watching the extra footage on the DVD's and seeing how things were done – actually being able to not only understand what they are explaining but being able to relay that story to my husband without stuttering or forgetting major details.

I have even been able to play some of the Harry Potter video games – which I thought was something I would only have fond memories of.

I know not everyone is a fan of the series, but everyone has something they love and enjoy, something that can help them heal. Find it! Find what works for you and embrace it. Use it to move forward, to get back some of your pre-injury skills, or to learn new ones. Have fun!

Recovery is a brutal and often solitary road and you deserve the best possible recovery.

You never know until you try just how magical using something you love can work to help you heal.

Meet Tobie-Lynn Andrade

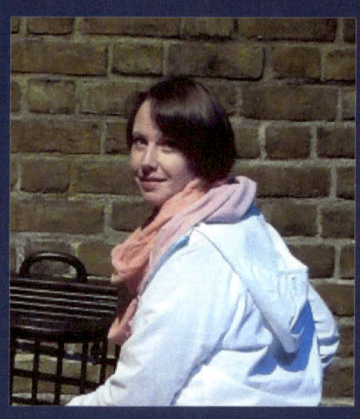

Tobie-Lynn is a lifelong fan of reading and an avid crafter, as well as a huge Harry Potter geek. She is recovering from a grade three concussion with front left lobe damage and post-concussion syndrome with seizures.

Tobie-Lynn is using natural medicines and methods to heal from her injuries, and the Harry Potter stories to help herself heal.

One of her greatest moments in life was going to England where the Harry Potter series was filmed and standing with her husband on the actual bridge used in the films.

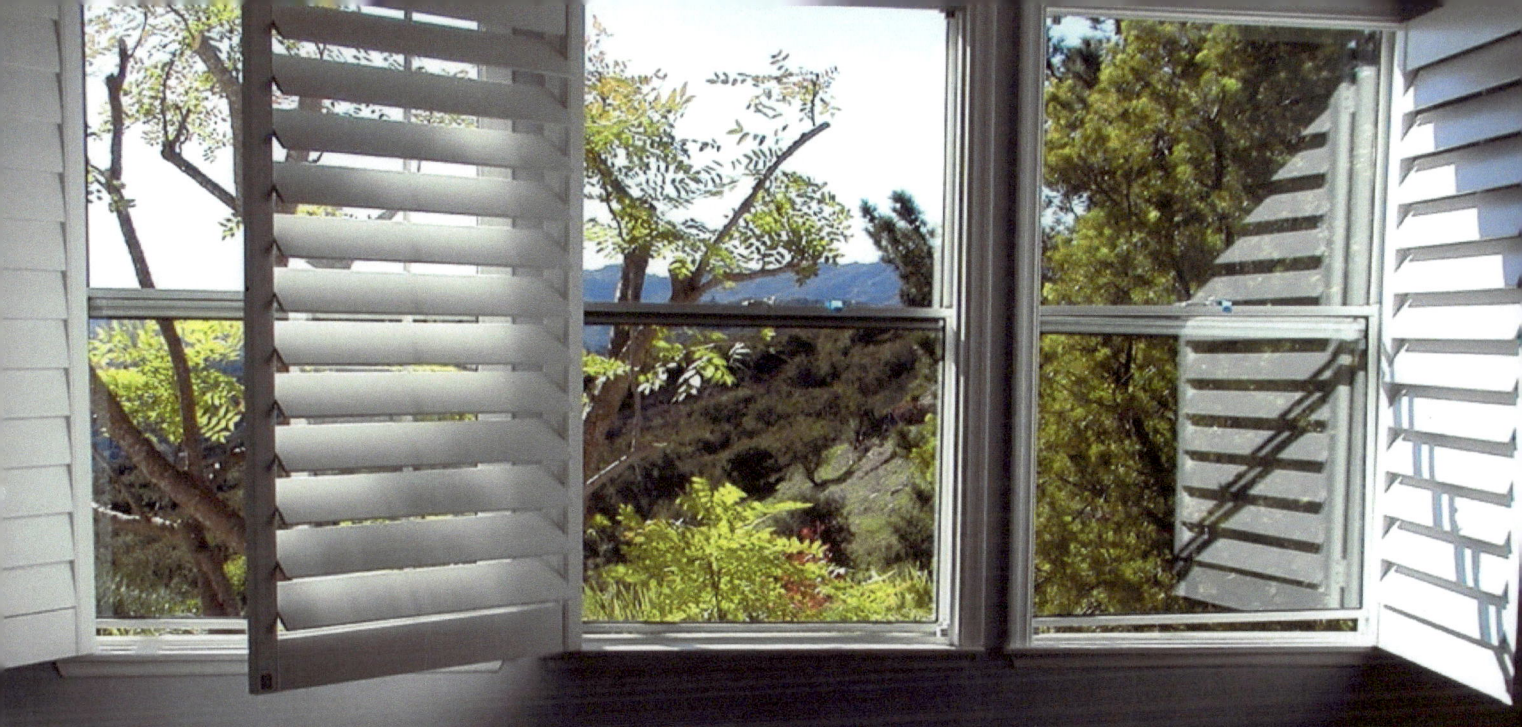

Colter's Story

By Mandi Seipel

Colter Pollock is an amazing, energetic, brave seven-year-old boy who suffered a Traumatic Brain Injury after a tragic fall from his second story bedroom window. On July 7, 2014, after a weekend of camping, the evening was supposed to be spent winding down but became our worst nightmare.

Five-year-old Colter was in a timeout in his bedroom after having poor behavior at the dinner table. At that time, his eight-year-old sister Jayden, and two-year-old brother Jaxon were playing in the backyard while I was cleaning up after supper. The sliding glass door was open, a slight breeze coming through and I could hear and see Jayden and Jaxon using their imaginations, playing away. Just as I was about to walk upstairs to talk to Colter about his manners at dinner time, the unimaginable happened.

I heard a loud crash that sounded like an egg cracking. Immediately, I ran outside to see Colter lifeless and blue, lying on his back on the concrete patio. Lying next to Colter was the window screen. Frantically, I urged my daughter to run and get help while I retrieved my phone and called 911. I was in such panic that I almost forget my password to unlock my phone and even contemplated what number to dial. When the responder answered, I yelled my address and repeated it twice. At about this time, Jayden came running back saying our neighbors were not home.

While on the phone with 911, my hands were shaking so badly that I couldn't find the pulse on Colter's wrist. What I did know is that he was turning blue and was not moving. Just as I was hearing the 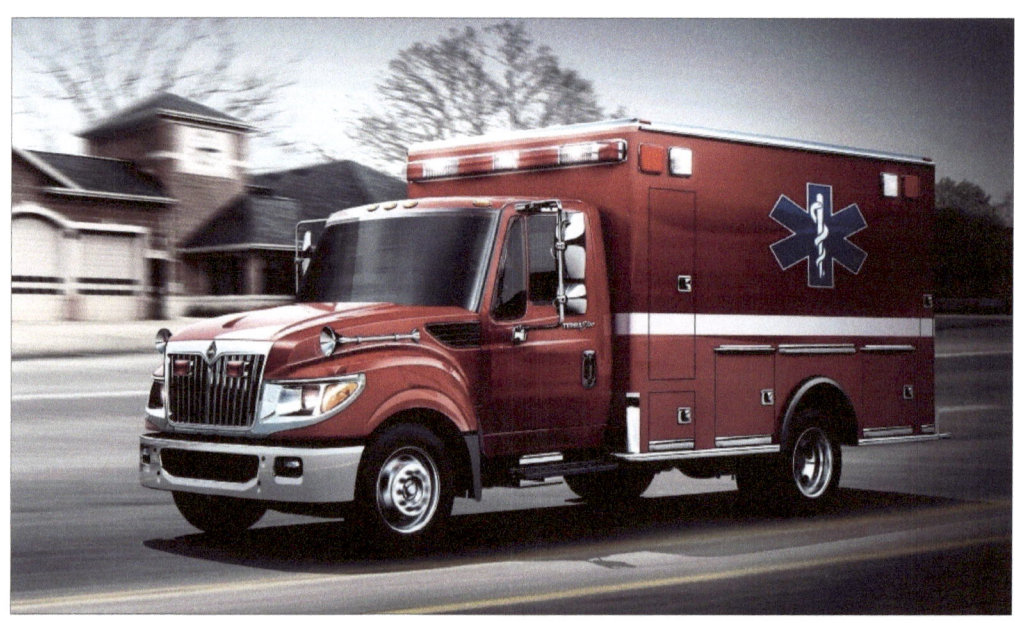 sirens, Jayden returned with our neighbor Ryan Ostrander, who happens to be an EMT. He calmly and quickly performed CPR on Colter and affirmed that he did have a faint pulse. Some days, it feels like it just happened yesterday… raw but almost dream-like.

Later at the ER, we learned that Colter had traumatic damage to his skull. His brain was swelling, there was a bleed and he also had fixed dilated pupils. However, I had no idea what a brain injury entailed. We would find out that Colter suffered a Severe Traumatic Brain Injury, along with a secondary diagnosis of left frontal temporal lobe contusion with a small subarachnoid hemorrhage.

After being life-flighted in a helicopter to Swedish Medical Center in Englewood, Colorado, I was told by his neurosurgeon Dr. Kimball, that Colter was a very sick boy and the chances of survival were slim. He explained that Colter would need a left frontotemporoparietal hemicraniectomy for subdural hematoma evacuation to relieve the swelling in his brain. The only glimpse of hope he gave me was when he said he had performed a craniotomy over 100 times and that he had not lost anyone yet. Signing consent papers stating that one of the outcomes was death left me both hopeless and ill.

Over the next 4 months, Colter's journey became a list of unknowns. Miraculously, he did not break or damage anything else. However, the questions were never ending: Will he survive? When will he open his eyes? When will I hear his voice? Will he have his memory? Would he walk? How would he be cognitively?

> *"Over the next 4 months, Colter's journey became a list of unknowns."*

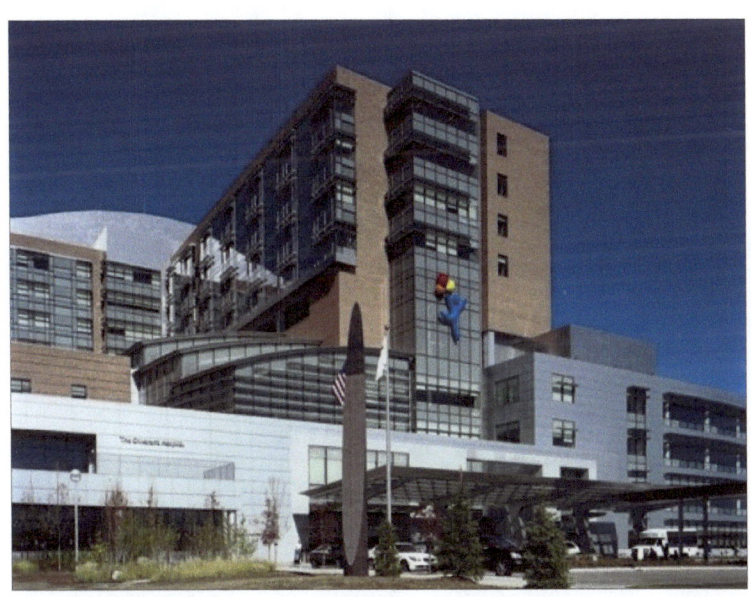

Colter spent three weeks at Swedish Medical Center then was transferred to the rehab unit of Children's Hospital in Colorado.

It was at Children's Hospital where Colter began learning all of life's simple, basic skills. We basically witnessed all of his life milestones for the second time.

During many moments, it felt like he would never be "normal" again. But, what I did not know then is that not only is TBI an invisible, uneducated injury, but that he would never 100% recover.

Colter is purely God's miracle. While Colter was in an induced coma, Dr. Kimball said that Colter's life will be a marathon. In the past two and a half years I often come back to the word, "marathon."

Colter has defied the odds in his journey thus far. This marathon has not been an easy race. We have hit a lot of bumps along the way and are still learning how we can pace him on his journey. One of the hardest parts of his injury is that he looks and appears to be normal, and it is easy for his behaviors to be misinterpreted. Hard days are hard, but we are blessed and very proud of his achievements.

Today, Colter is a determined seven-year-old, first-grade boy who loves sports, is great at math and reading, and plans to grow up working with animals.

Although Colter is defeating the odds, it's important to note that his journey of healing has not been an easy one. He has challenges and struggles that include his eyesight, sensitivity to light, perseveration, impulsiveness, safety awareness, headaches, and fatigue.

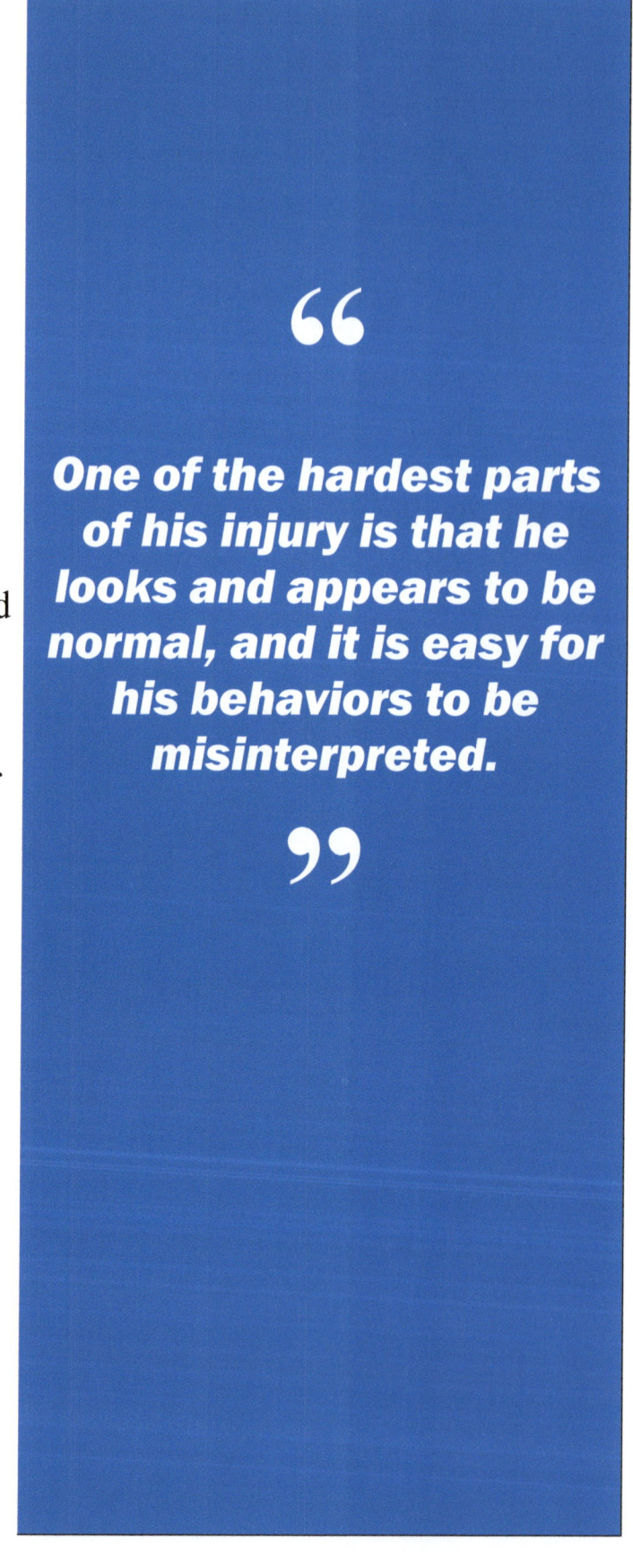

One of the hardest parts of his injury is that he looks and appears to be normal, and it is easy for his behaviors to be misinterpreted.

These are not closed chapters, but ones that are real to the effects of a Traumatic Brain Injury. We continue to not only advocate for window fall prevention but also raise awareness about brain injuries and preventable accidents.

It is our hope that we can prevent these types of accidents from happening to other children and families.

EDITOR'S NOTE:

April is Window Fall Prevention Month. For information about raising safety and awareness in your home and community, visit www.stopat4.com.

To follow Colter's story, visit his Facebook page: I Believe in Colter.

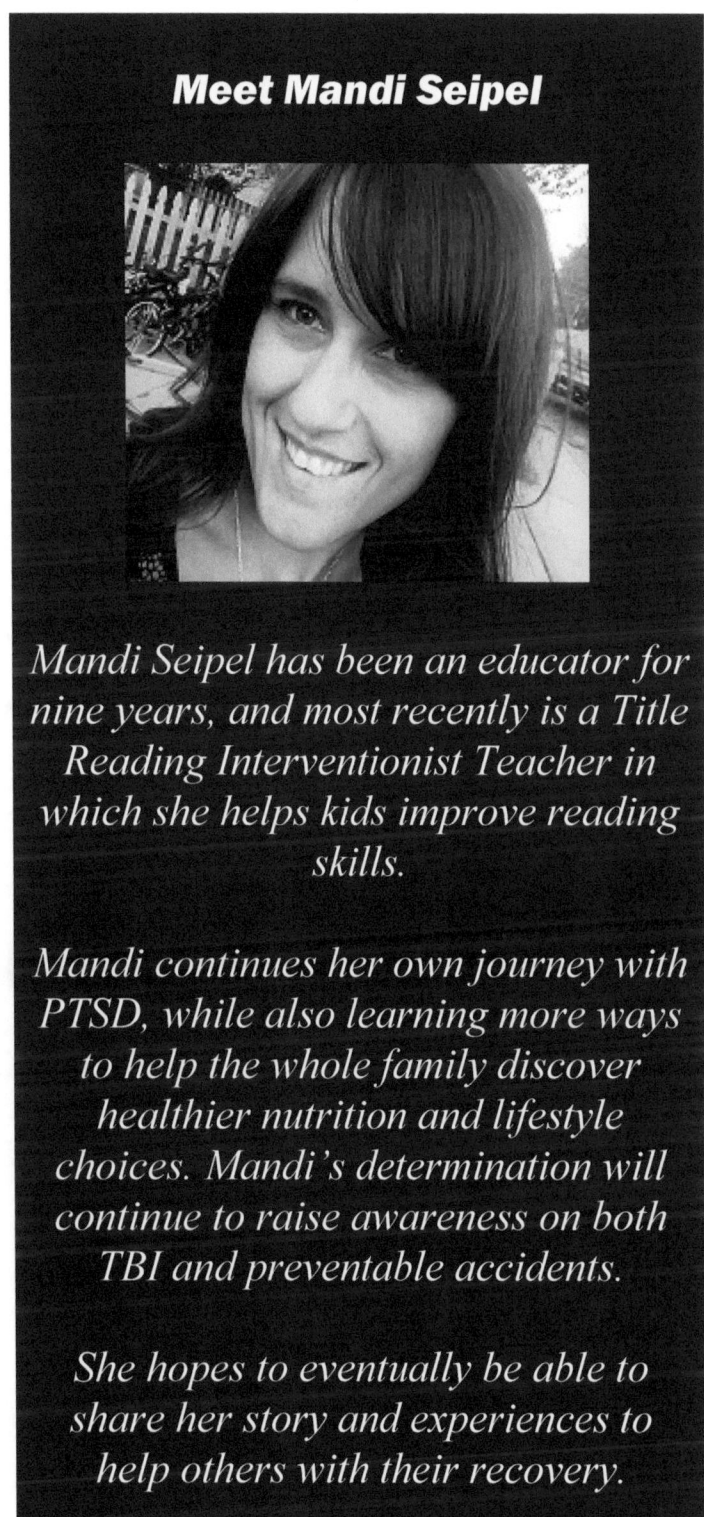

Meet Mandi Seipel

Mandi Seipel has been an educator for nine years, and most recently is a Title Reading Interventionist Teacher in which she helps kids improve reading skills.

Mandi continues her own journey with PTSD, while also learning more ways to help the whole family discover healthier nutrition and lifestyle choices. Mandi's determination will continue to raise awareness on both TBI and preventable accidents.

She hopes to eventually be able to share her story and experiences to help others with their recovery.

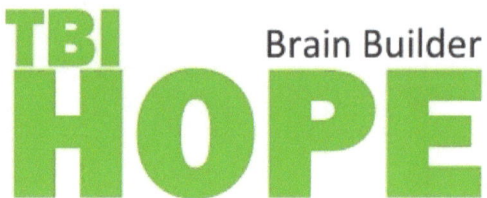

Brain Builder

Word Search

```
C T A N O R U E N C Y B
L O T C M J N N I Y R R
Y G N J Q P Z T D A T X
T P Z C M U A L I R K T
E V P Y U M I N H O P E
D K P Y U S B R N Q L Q
D R O A D L S T E Y K J
J J R R J V I I Q D T D
L T X M T J R B O L D D
N Q V Y T S M T L N M D
```

Concussion	Stroke
Brain	Traumatic
Neuron	Mri
Hope	Acquired

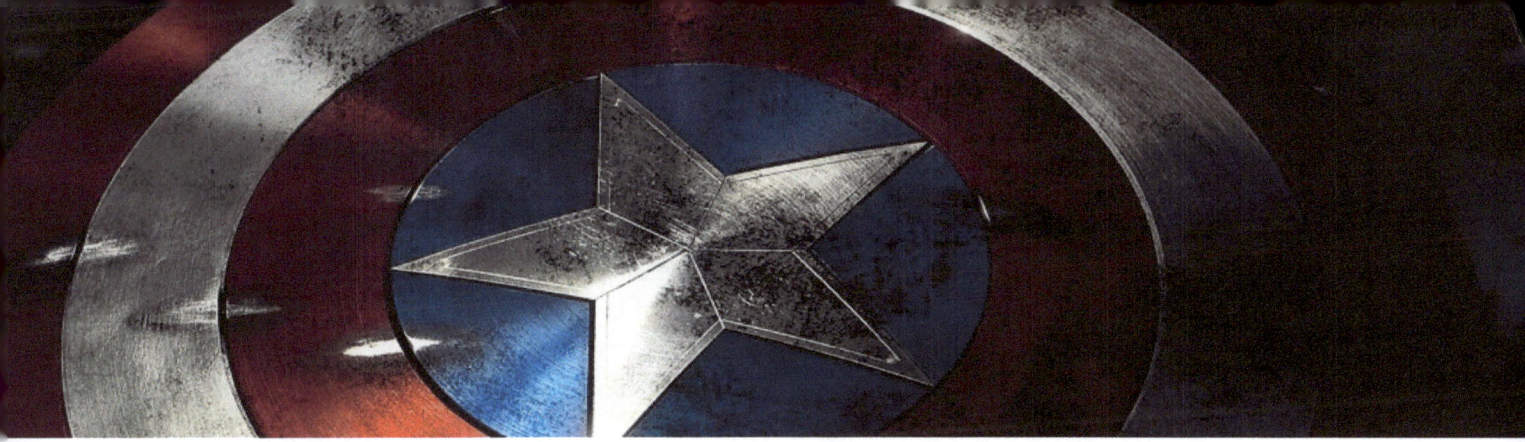

TBI - To Become Invincible

By Nick Dennen

I was born on Wednesday, April 26, 1978, but my life actually began on Sunday, September 27, 1998. At age 20, I experienced a re-birth, a renewal of life. I was born again, not only in the sense of accepting God into my life, but it was when I discovered my purpose. I had lived 7,459 days not knowing who I was or what I was supposed to do with my life. Mark Twain has said, "The two most important days in your life are the day you are born and the day you find out why."

My "why" arrived in the form of an inspiring message borne from a 35-foot fall, a near drowning, and a two-year rehabilitation. I was at an after-game party drinking with my teammates; I was underage. The party was "busted." I don't remember that night, or the week before. All I know is that a police officer who was patrolling wanted to investigate what I was doing walking alone at 2:38am, and I was chased by his police dog. It's assumed that I was trying to escape the dog and fell off a cliff.

I was unconscious for roughly two months; death was near. My actual time in the coma is questionable however. Even when my eyes opened, I was still completely out of it. I couldn't do anything other than simply lie there. So many people can relate to this pain. Brain injury affects different people in different ways; however, what we share in rehab experience is comparable. Having to relearn certain skills like walking, talking, writing, feeding oneself, brushing one's teeth, or more practical strengths like shopping, organizing data, and making calls to a repair company, do not come easy. In fact, they are practically impossible.

But with physical therapy, occupational therapy, and speech therapy, a person can evolve and become human again. By enduring a TBI, it erases the young person who was once there, the "Old Nick," and begins to construct the new individual who is here now, the "New Nick!" Rebuilding is the key. Yes, you will never be who you were, but with the right guidance, you can change who you'll become.

My entire right side was paralyzed for months. I lost over forty pounds in a matter of a couple months. I was tube fed. I wore diapers. I had to drink thickened liquids. I ate beets, and I hate that disgusting vegetable. I had

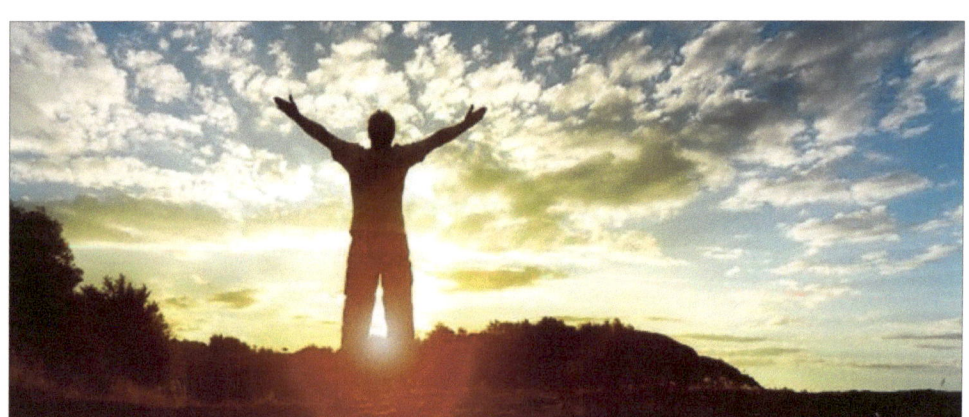

slurred speech. I had chest tubes. I still have a bald spot on the back of my head showing where my hair fell out. I have a scar on the middle of my throat where the trach was. This is a daily reminder of when life tried (key word here is "tried") to beat me down. My family went through hell not knowing if I would ever get to a point where I could write this story.

What is most unfortunate is how "easy" the media and/or people in general make a recovery from a brain injury seem to be. It does not happen overnight. My rehabilitation took roughly two years, but I can honestly say that it took much longer than that. The "experts" say that recovery from a brain injury is a two-year process. I agree, I was able to start walking, begin to talk and perform certain tasks, and go back to school after a couple years, but I feel that it takes much longer than two years to rebuild and enhance the life that was stolen.

So much of what we have gone through can help other people.

There is a saying that it takes ten years to become an overnight success. This seems to be more accurate. It also says it takes 10,000 hours to become an expert on something—this averages out to be 20 hours a week for 10 years.

With a TBI, this is something we all have "blood memory" of. We have owned every experience, every setback, every loss, every victory, and every lesson we wish we wouldn't have had to learn. We own the pain of our family and friends. So, I think it would be fair to say that based on these statistics, all of us who experienced our TBI, can be regarded as "experts" on brain injury approximately 417 days after our brains were damaged. Pretty cool, huh?

The critics would disagree. They don't want us to succeed. They don't want us to share our life experience for the greater good. So much of what we have gone through can help other people. So much of our lives can give hope to somebody else. It is more than just surviving a brain injury; it is thriving because of the brain injury.

It is a way to enhance the healing and develop a stronger version of yourself. The TBI may have ripped our worlds to shreds, but it can be pieced back together through faith, hope, and love.

It is what we experience that can change a life. It is our stories that give strength to an important cause. It is our stories that allow others to share theirs. And it is how we think of our traumatic brain injury that defines us.

TBI is defined as Traumatic Brain Injury. After receiving mine, I have come to realize that TBI has multiple meanings.

1. TBI: To Believe in the Impossible.
2. TBI: To Baffle the Imagination.
3. TBI: To see Beyond the Individual.
4. TBI: To Become Invincible.

David A. Grant, speaker and founder of *TBI Hope & Inspiration*, believes TBI means "To Be Inspired." We all need to be inspired. A TBI truly is more than just a traumatic brain injury. It is a life-changing event which tests our strengths, while highlighting our weaknesses. It ultimately comes down to either seeing your glass half-empty, or seeing it as half-full.

> *"It ultimately comes down to either seeing your glass half-empty, or seeing it as half-full."*

Initially, I only saw all the things I had lost—the abilities, the future, the life—and wasn't willing to see the things I had won—the new abilities, the new future, the new life. Was it the brain injury preventing me from seeing the bigger picture? Perhaps.

I thought my life was over; I didn't think I was good enough. I thought my brain injury had won. This is all nonsense. It is my hope that reading about my experience will change your perspective, and give you the hope necessary to move forward.

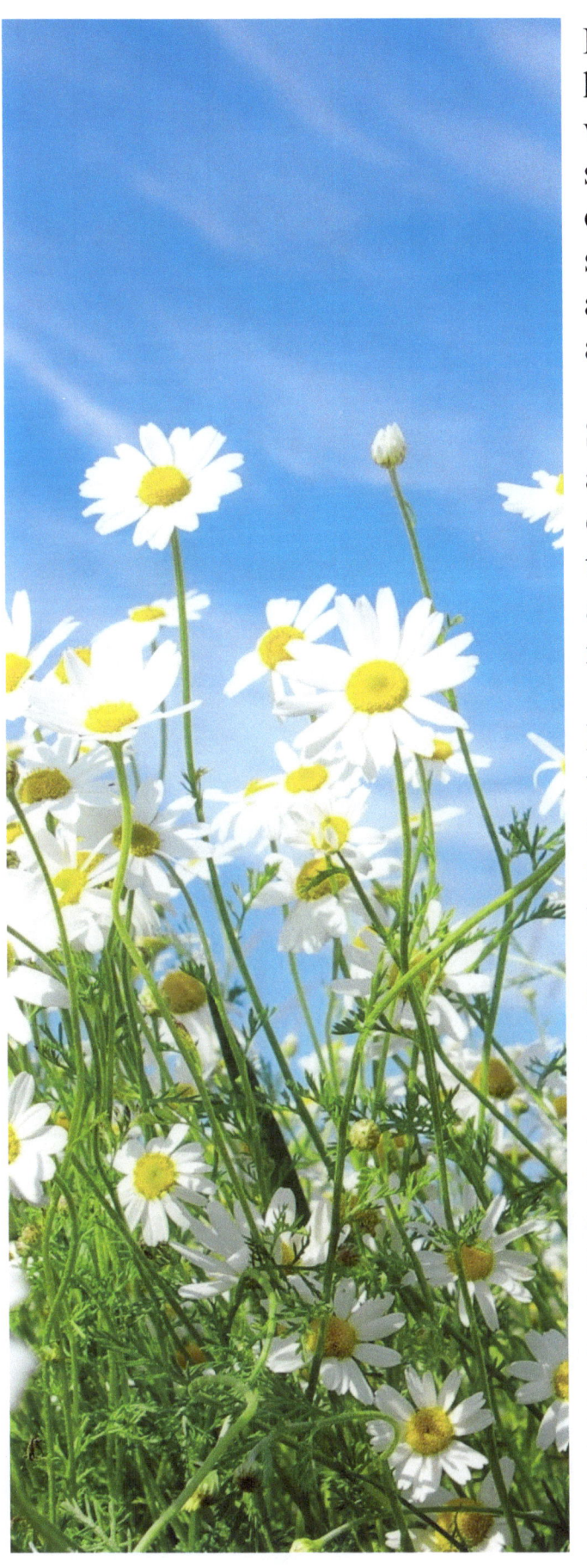

My balance is off, and I walk with kind of a slight limp at times, but I am walking. When I am tired, my speech seems to be a little delayed (probably only to me), but I am talking. My right side is still weaker than my left, but I am still able to work out like a house afire at the gym.

So much of what we all experience after enduring a brain injury are experiences that do hold the potential to benefit us. I guess it comes down to a matter of perspective, where many of my limitations are self-imposed.

Did I ever think I would go through what I had? Heck no! This was something that always happened to somebody else. But once I came to terms with where I was, I was able to see "why" I had been given this knowledge or opportunity, and what I was supposed to do with it.

My former theology professor taught me a theory he developed years ago called The Dorito Principle. A Dorito has three sides. The first side suggests we "Seek to thrive." We can overcome our pains and enhance our life. The second side says, "Seek to love and be loved." We must love others as we love ourselves.

And the third side says, "To live for the common good!"

Our life's purpose is to make a positive difference in the world. It is never about "us," rather it is about "them," and helping others. I had to redefine TBI.

It is so important to always remember that we are part of something bigger than ourselves. We can make a difference in the world. It's important to remember all the things that we are so extremely fortunate to have.

Always recognize that people have feelings—life is too short to hold a grudge—and never be ashamed for the person you are and everything you stand for. Every person matters, and every single life is sacred and deals with its own yesterdays, tomorrows, and todays.

Remember that your attitude will either lift you up or bring you down, so please make the choice to live your best life now.

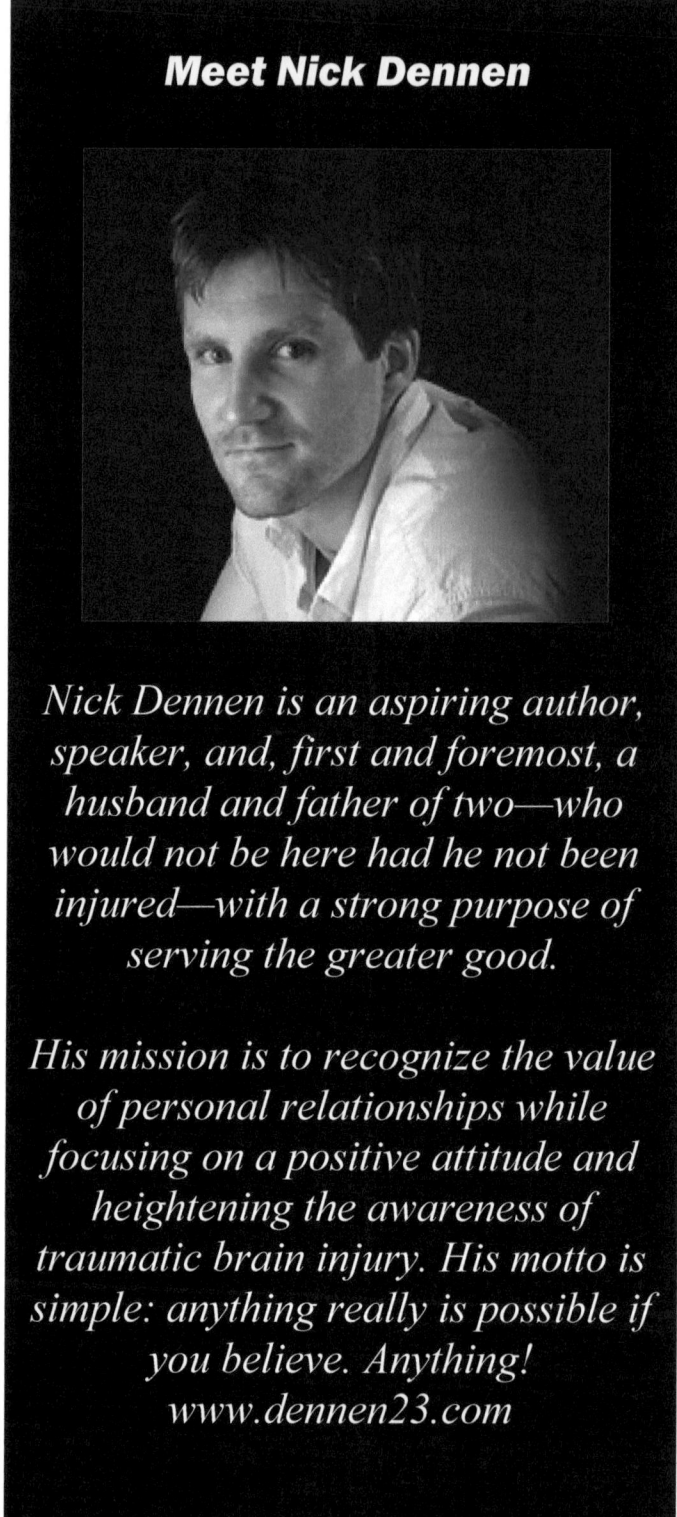

Meet Nick Dennen

Nick Dennen is an aspiring author, speaker, and, first and foremost, a husband and father of two—who would not be here had he not been injured—with a strong purpose of serving the greater good.

His mission is to recognize the value of personal relationships while focusing on a positive attitude and heightening the awareness of traumatic brain injury. His motto is simple: anything really is possible if you believe. Anything!
www.dennen23.com

Injured, A Poetic Tribute

By Molly Dorhauer

I know it's been awhile,
the injury began ages ago,
but when the 'bad' days
still creep along,
please, I beg,
be patient.
There are times before the Sun
chooses to peak over my horizon,
and no one has told me
what I should be;
it is only then that I know,
I am.
Before job offers
of impossibilities
knock upon my door,
and before I forget which month time
has chosen it to be,
I can breathe,
and even dream
Of a life where memories
aren't a collected, disheveled mess
lost somewhere between
what ifs and
chances mistaken.
My heart still feels cheated
from all of the lessons relearned
but it beats stronger from necessity,
knowing
that there is more to me.

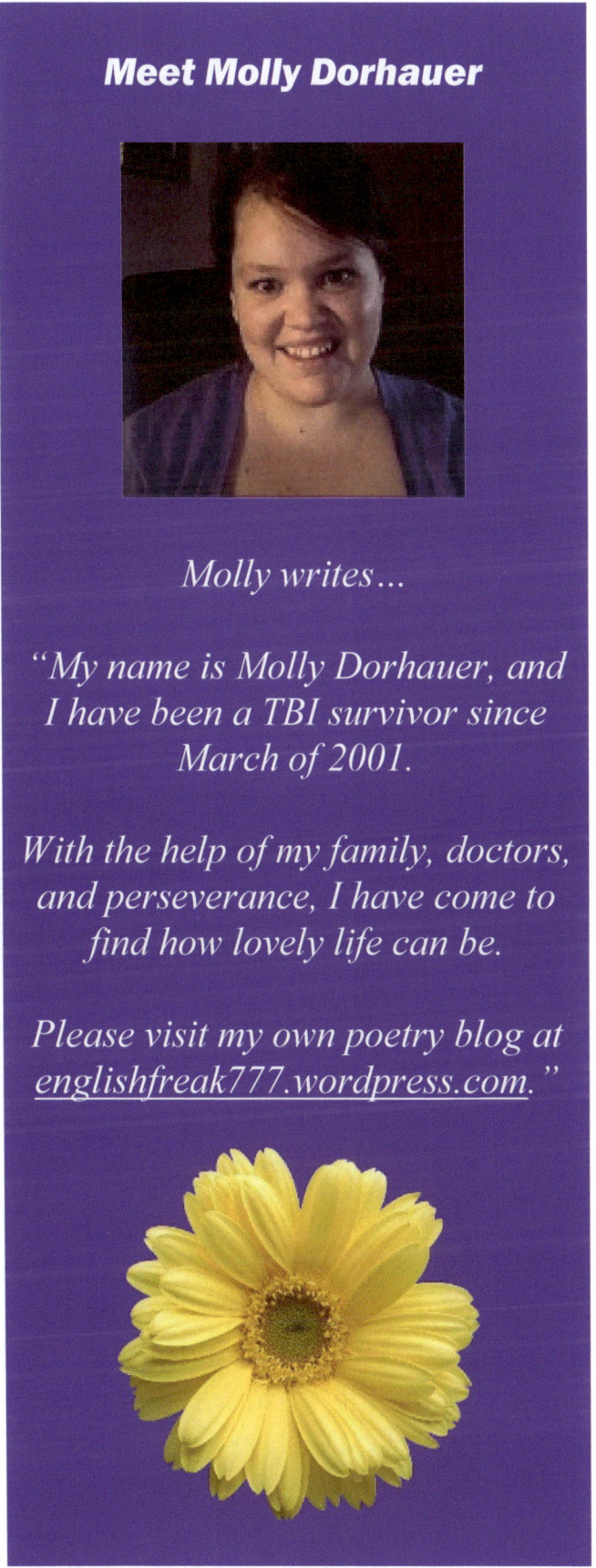

Meet Molly Dorhauer

Molly writes...

"My name is Molly Dorhauer, and I have been a TBI survivor since March of 2001.

With the help of my family, doctors, and perseverance, I have come to find how lovely life can be.

Please visit my own poetry blog at englishfreak777.wordpress.com."

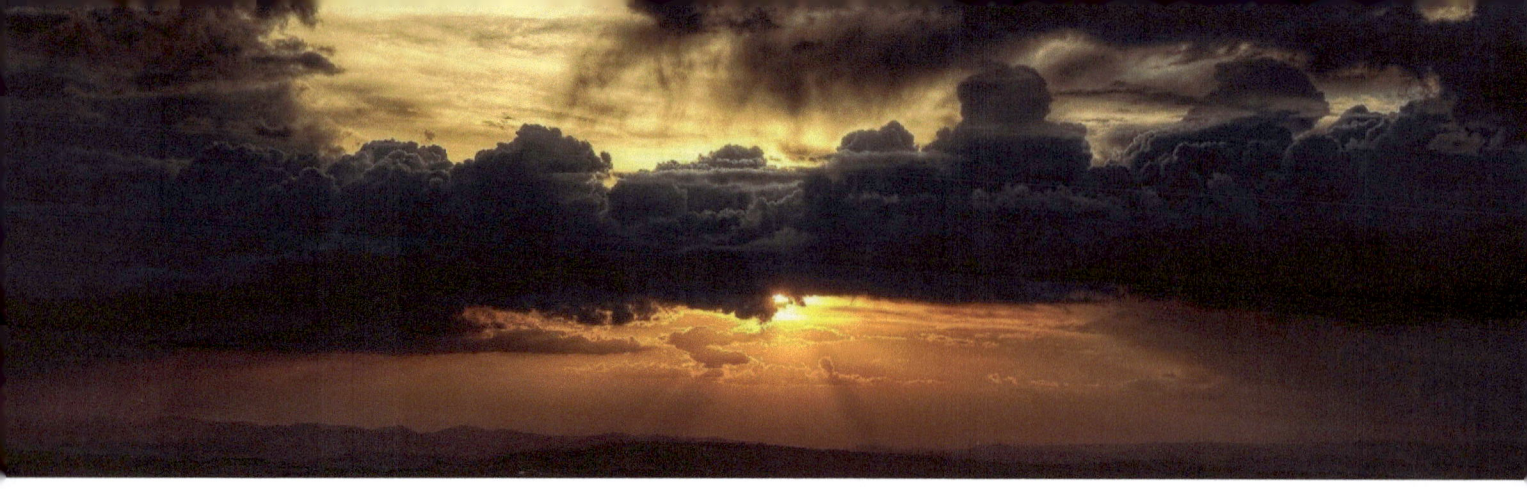

How do I Win the War?

By Nancy Bauser

How do I win the war against my problems?

I've learned that I must accept what I absolutely cannot do before I will allow myself to begin to learn the skills necessary to do what I want. Then, I must realize that every day and every task is different. Just because I'm able to do something today, at a particular time, doesn't mean that I'll be able to repeat that behavior on another day or at another time.

Remember that trauma, injury, disability or illness are the problems. Is it worth the struggle to try to recover? I say, YES, it is. I accept myself with all my limitations! I always try to do the best that I can with what I've got.

Making progress is simple, but it certainly isn't easy. It requires commitment and a sustained determination to overcome obstacles and attain goals. My life has taught me that I was not singled out for the terrible misfortunes that I've experienced. That awareness doesn't eliminate or minimize my problems, but it does reduce the suffering that comes from struggling against the unfortunate facts of my life.

I have problems with my memory and making good judgments. I forget lots of things. I put something somewhere and then forget where I put it. I miss appointments, or I forget to do things that I know I want to do. I get easily confused and reacting immediately simply cannot be done.

What do I do? I need to have a plan.

Mine is three steps:

First, it's best to confront rather than avoid the difficulties created by my trauma, injury, disability or illness.

Next, I must think of myself as having a battle with the deficits created by problems.

Lastly, if I am ignorant of my difficulties, I will be unable to avoid or reduce my own suffering.

I wish things were different, but they're not. All I can do is the best that I can - and like myself in the process.

When I familiarize myself with the difficulties that might occur, my distress about life with all my problems seems to be reduced, as well as my fear and anxiety.

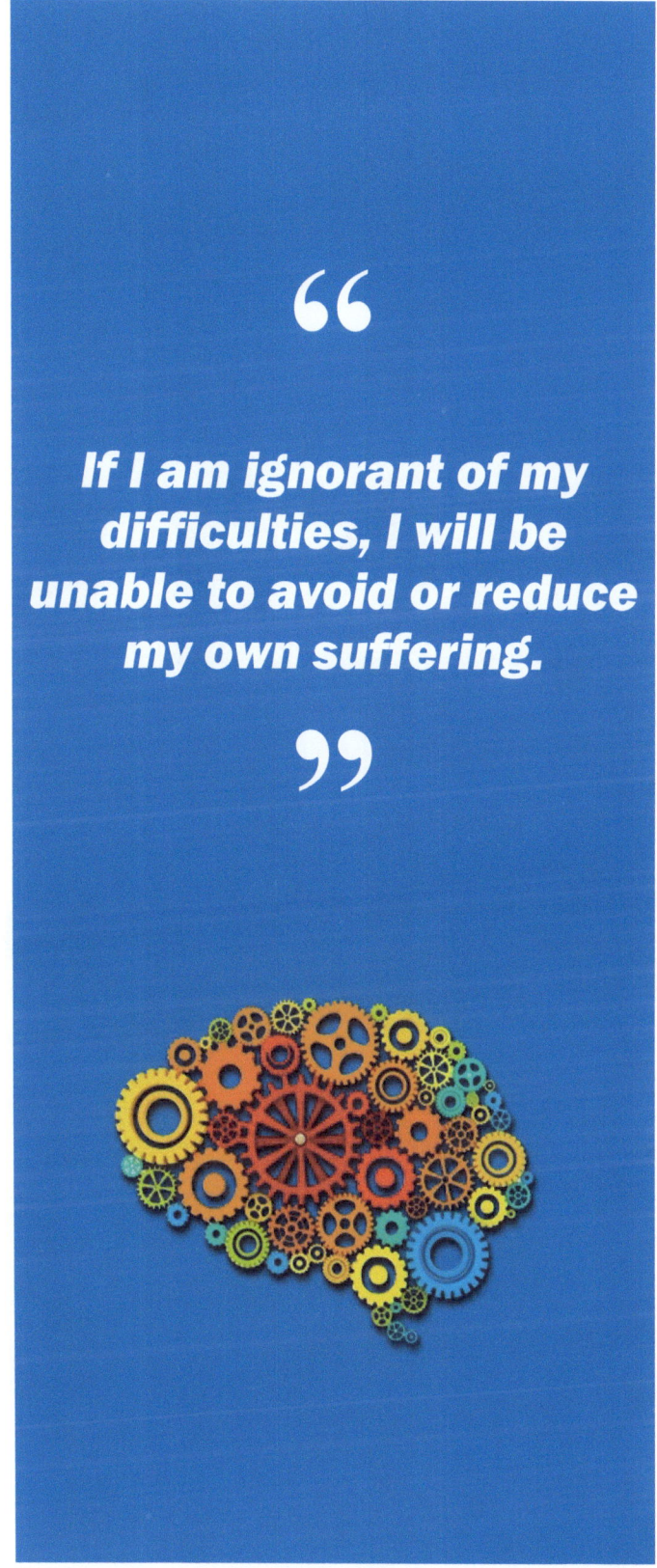

"

If I am ignorant of my difficulties, I will be unable to avoid or reduce my own suffering.

"

Meet Nancy Bauser

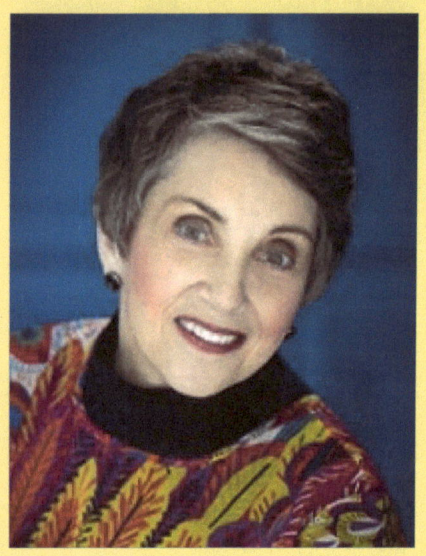

Nancy Bauser is a disability life coach. Over forty-three years ago – in 1971, Nancy sustained a severe closed head/brain stem injury while attending undergraduate school.

A longtime resident of Bloomfield Hills, MI, Nancy maintains an active profile in the community and supports organizations that benefit healthcare recipients.

In her spare time, Nancy's interests include writing, exercising, long distance walking and being with friends and family. You can read more of Nancy's work at www.survivoracceptance.com.

When I no longer need to be afraid of what might happen, I'm able to better prepare for the options or success strategies that I must use.

To make changes, I need goals. I recognize my difficulties in the here and now. When creating genuine change, I must make a sustained effort. My experiences have taught me that it takes time and effort to modify behavior.

One statement that I often repeat to myself is, Recovery is not only Making Progress; it is Taking Just One Step! I always need to remember that it doesn't matter where I start. Doing anything to make my life better is Making Progress.

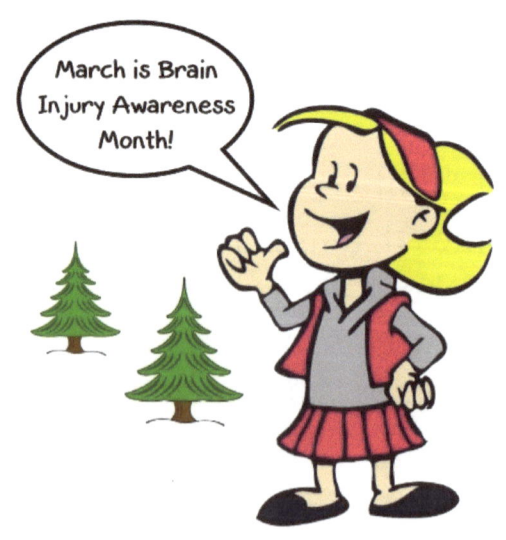

March is Brain Injury Awareness Month!

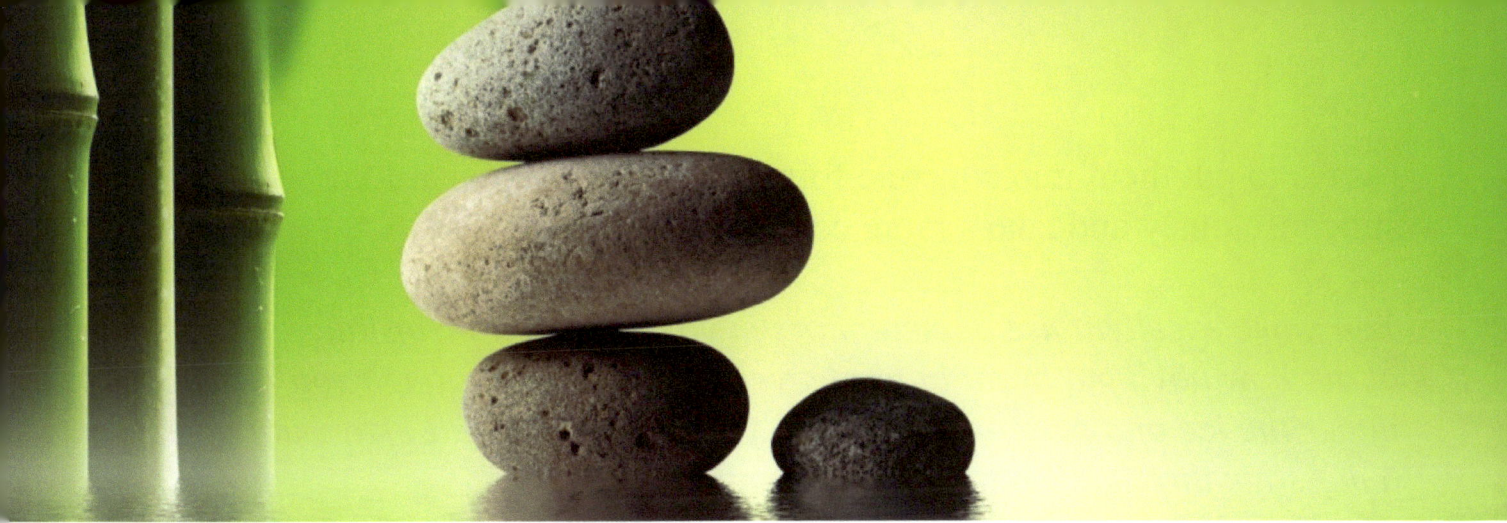

My Post-TBI Life
An Interview with Mike Strand

In 1999, Mike Strand began writing short essays about living with brain injury and the lessons he has learned. He began writing to help others understand their own brain injuries but soon found that his own self-understanding was growing too. Now his essays have been collected in *Meditations on Brain* Injury from Lash and Associates, small but powerful books valuable to anyone who wants to learn more about living with an injured brain.

Did you write before your brain injury?

No. I considered myself a writer, but like a lot of people who say that, hadn't actually written.

Do you keep a journal?

No. My alternative to journaling is to write these essays. I originally wrote them to help others, but they helped me. I take my vague notions and use the essays to put them into concrete form. They spell out what I know subconsciously and take a more coherent form.

You make excellent use of metaphors in your essays. For instance, there's one about how having a brain injury leaves you feeling as though you're trapped under the ice of a frozen lake, where, you write, "I'm still okay but I can't get a message through." Why do you use metaphors?

It's pretty effortless for me to make these metaphors. Especially with brain injury, if you're telling people "It's like…" it makes it easier for them to get it. With writing, I can come up with good metaphors. I can occasionally make them up in conversation, but it usually takes extra time, which is not a luxury I have when talking to people.

> *"Take stock of what you've got, look at where you want to go, and start working toward it."*

You write that "Wellness isn't just a catchy phrase for me, but a moral imperative." That's an intriguing statement. Please explain why this is true for you.

For a lot of people, "wellness" is a generic term meaning, "I want to feel healthy." For me, it's a much more intentional step-by-step process. Successful people say you have to have a plan—write it down. So after a brain injury, you have to write it down, what you want to accomplish.

Why do you say "post-TBI" rather than "recovery"?

Just saying "recovery" is too limiting and not really accurate. Post-TBI, you're not even going in the same direction, it's like after your accident your car was facing another direction, and driving straight back is never going to get you where you were. You have to find acceptance. If you're trying to recover, you're not accepting. Recovery is impossible because you're changed. Take stock of what you've got, look at where you want to go, and start working toward it.

In the "About the Author" section in the book, you write about yourself, "His life before his brain injury was spent consistently under-achieving based on his abilities, and over-questioning in lieu of accomplishing. Brain injury recovery was the challenge that finally lit a spark in his soul and dared him to do better." That's very honest and beautiful.

I cobbled that together bit by bit. I looked at what my strengths are and how has brain injury changed me. Before, I used foolishness in lieu of accomplishing. I didn't have that luxury after the brain injury.

I like that you say in one of your essays, "Who you are is a dynamic process." Please explain, especially in terms of post-TBI.

It's because so often with TBI, especially early on, you feel like you have so far to go. So you have to accept that you're growing and changing at all times. If you define yourself in a static sense, it's self-defeating. You need to look beyond "Who am I?" to "Who am I becoming?"

You write, "Brain injury is an opportunity to design yourself all over again." How have you done that?

I wouldn't have said that early on. But I remember a conversation about what I would do if I had to do it all over again—I've been given that opportunity, whether I like it or not. So how do I choose to view this? I've done all these things because of my brain injury.

One change that happened for you post-TBI is that your heart compensated for your brain, as you describe it. How so?

Because before the accident I considered myself very intellectual, which made me dismissive of others. Since the brain injury, I don't feel that way. I have received such kindnesses, and if you're a human being, you reflect that back. I began seeing the world in a kinder light. I had to. I needed there to be warmth and friendliness. And I have no regrets.

You write about having a purpose in life after a TBI. Please talk about purpose and what it means to you now.

It goes hand-in-hand with what is the meaning of life. Why should I get out of bed? I see now why people who talk about purpose talk about helping others. If you're only doing something for your own personal gain, it's hard for that to feel fulfilling. The cool thing about finding purpose in your life—and it's almost always when you're giving—is that it gets your focus off yourself. Helping others takes the focus off ourselves.

Is there anything else you would like to add?

Reading this interview you might get the impression that I'm a pretty driven individual, and in some respects I am, but the things I say and the things I write are ideals to which I strive, frequently unsuccessfully. Writing essays, like journaling, helps me keep my focus and achieve my personal goals.

Meet Mike Strand

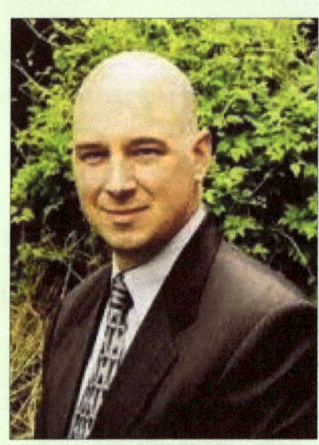

Mike Strand and his wife Linda have been married over 25 years and have known each other since they were kids.

In January of 1989, six months before their wedding, Mike was hit by a semi-truck as he drove home from work.

Mike has written three books of essays on brain injury that are available from Lash Publishing.

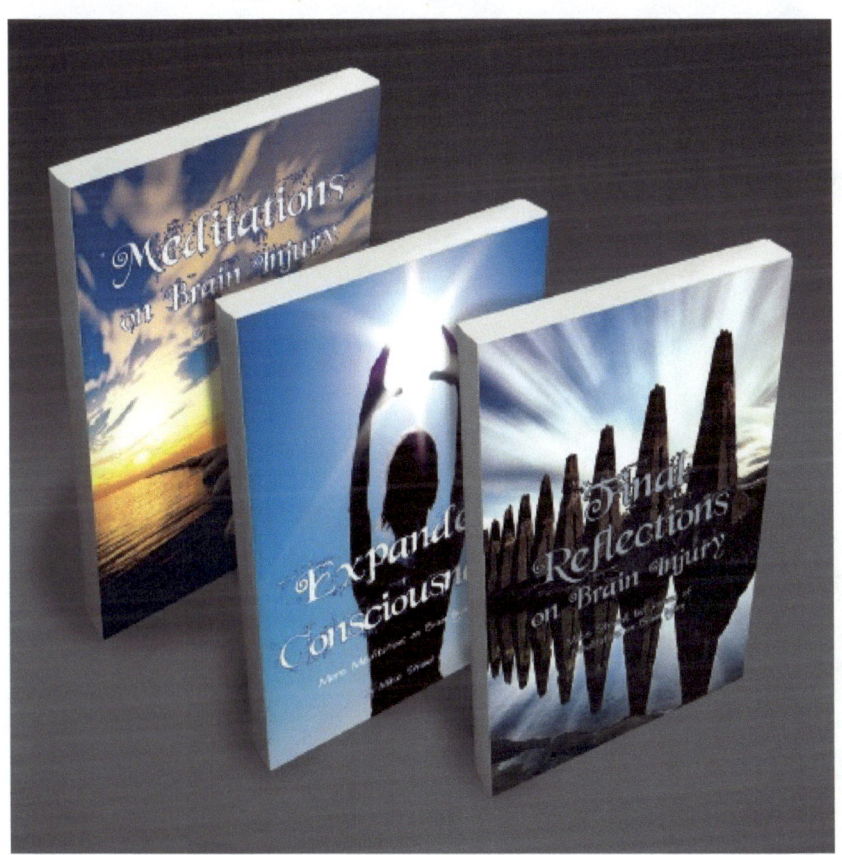

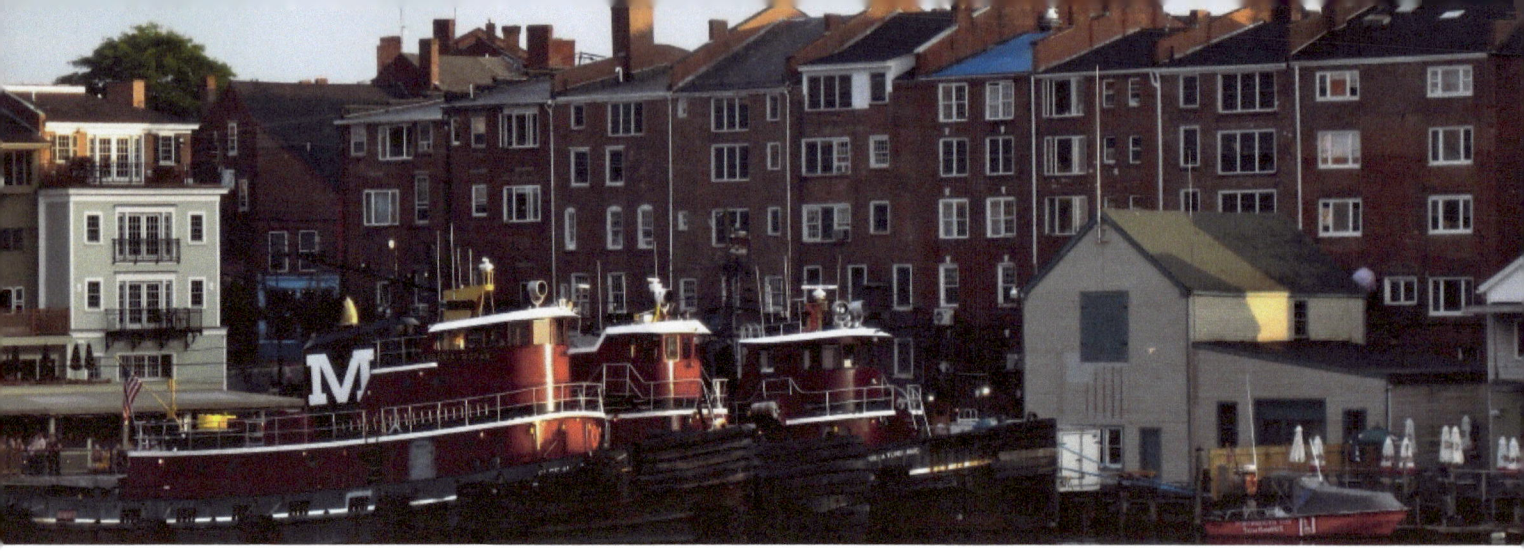

Taking that Small First Step

By Ralph Poland

On November 3rd, 2006 I went to the emergency room of York Hospital. Hours later, I suffered a heart attack. Then, I was transported to Portsmouth Regional Hospital to undergo open heart surgery. Due to complications, I was then transported to Tuft's Medical Center in Boston, Massachusetts where they re-performed the surgery. During the second operation, I suffered two debilitating strokes, which landed me in a coma for the next two and a half weeks.

During my coma, there were times of hearing strange voices talking about cabbage. Then, much later in my recovery I learned that cabbage is a medical term which means: [CABG "Coronary, Artery, Bypass, Graft"]

I came out of my coma shortly after being transported back to Portsmouth Regional Hospital, and discovered I had no feeling below my knees, elbows, nor use of my hands, as well as being unable to speak, finding myself in a kind of vegetative state. I was left only to peer out into the limited world around me. My whole body felt foreign to me and, even my thoughts were a hopelessly jumbled mess, I was surprised that it was almost Thanksgiving Day.

Then, one day as my two neurologists were leaving, one of them posed by my bed just long enough to say: "You'll be lucky if you are confined to a wheelchair for the rest of your life."

At some point, I realized that I needed to try to only think positive thoughts. I felt I had to try to put a positive spin on things because I couldn't afford to allow my mind to discourage me from even trying. I finally came up with simply adding 'Yet' at the end of my 'can't'. For example, my self-talk became "I can't do it yet," from that moment on.

Meanwhile, after five weeks in Portsmouth, I was moved to New England Rehab, in Portland Maine. There I began intensive Physical, Occupational, and Speech Therapies. When I first arrived, I couldn't feed myself and had to continue to be lifted in and out of bed by a lift that was bolted to the ceiling.

After many OT sessions, my therapist had me try to support myself enough to stand with the use of a walker. One day while having me do this exercise (feeling that I could confide in him), I told him that I wanted him to help me walk again.

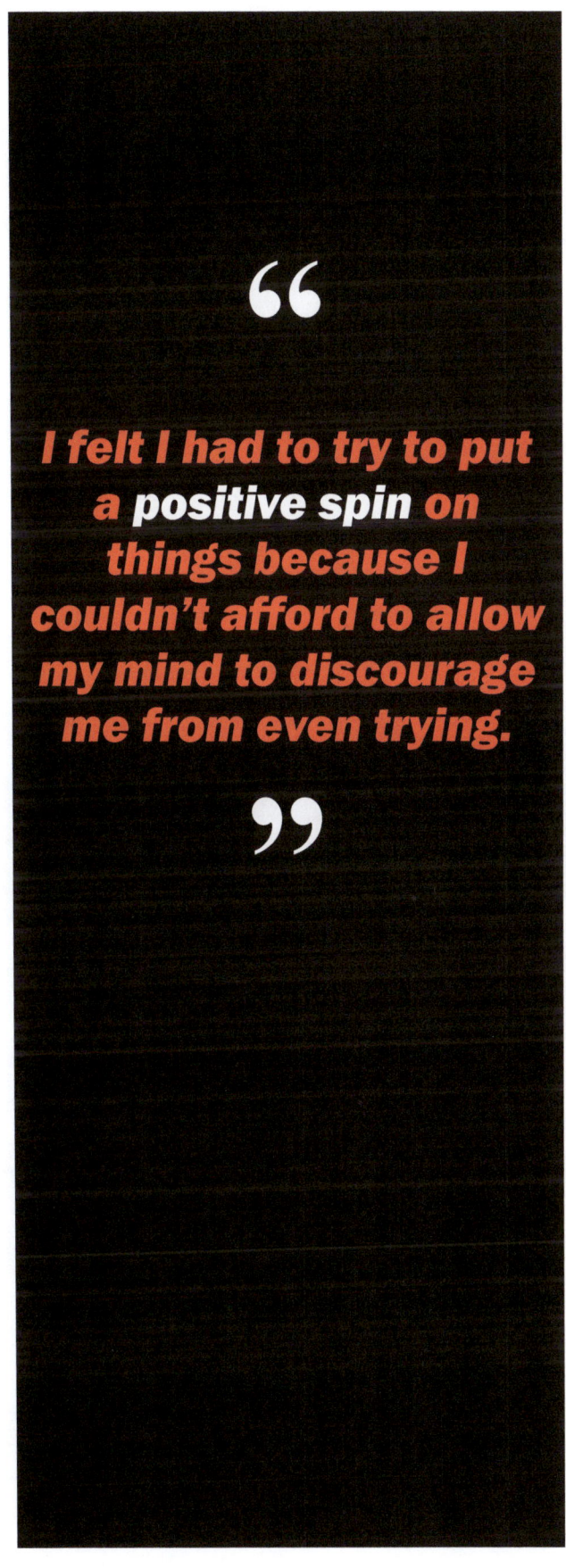

"
I felt I had to try to put a positive spin on things because I couldn't afford to allow my mind to discourage me from even trying.
"

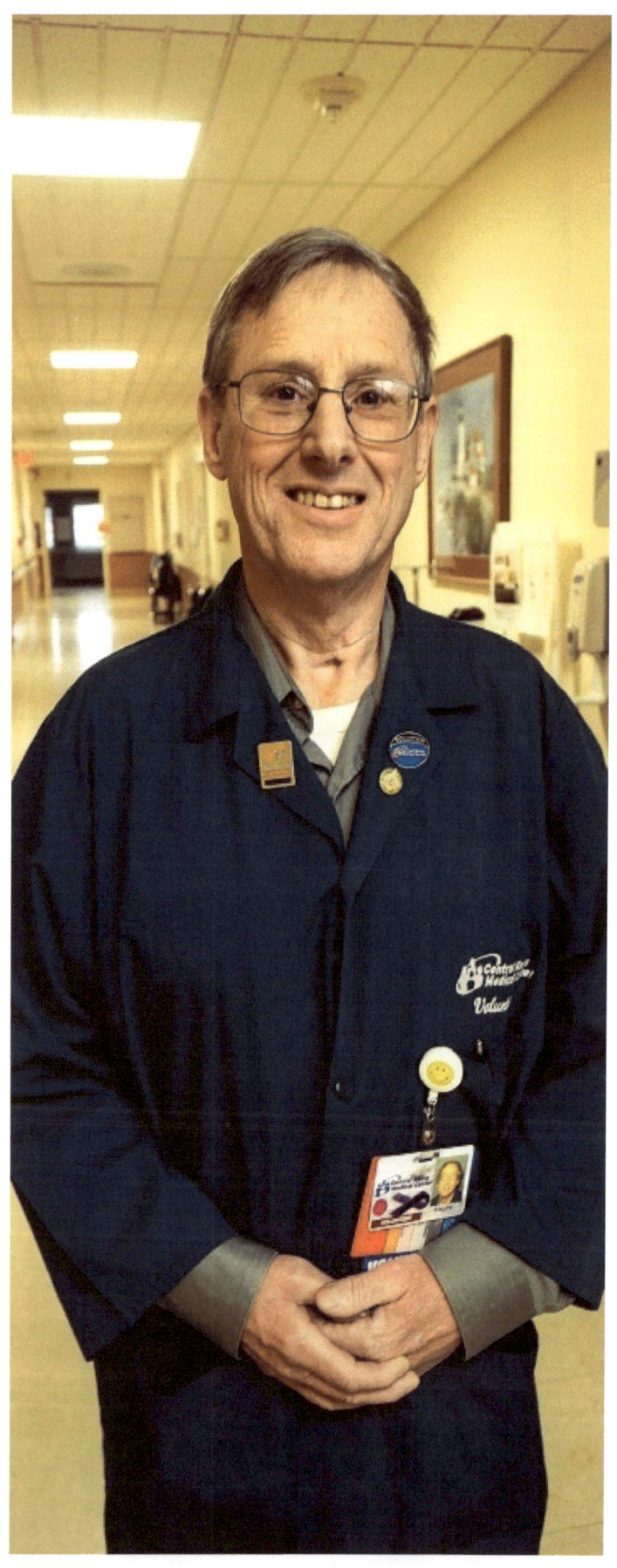

He replied, "I understand that you have no feeling below your knees, is that right?" I answered yes! Then he said, "Because you have no feeling in your lower legs, you wouldn't be able to learn to walk again." I was devastated when hearing that so I asked him to do me a favor.

First, I asked him to let me know when my left foot was firmly planted on the floor, indicating that my right foot was ready to take a step. He agreed. Then, I asked him to do the same with my right foot. Once he did, he asked, "What was that about?" I told him that each time I had made a mental note of how each upper leg felt, and now I am ready to walk! He replied, "You are determined to walk?" I answered "yes!" He then said, "Well, not today! We're at the end of this session and you are well spent. But, if you are so determined to try, then at some point we can try again."

About a week later, while my OT was wheeling me out through my room, he asked if I still wanted to try to walk. Of course I said yes! So, he stopped my wheel chair at the doorway of my room, then he placed my walker in front of me and said, "We'll try it right here."

I struggled very hard to slowly take the first small step. Then after a short pause, I continued with the next step. Due to being exhausted, I let myself drop back into my wheelchair. I heard my OT mutter, "Boy, you are determined!"

By the time I was discharged, I could walk one hundred feet with the use of my walker, before tiring.

Through Northern New England Goodwill's Neuro Rehab services, I was assigned to two PT's. Over time they tried introducing me to using every assistive device in their arsenal. One day while I was (again) trying to use a cane, that PT and I passed my other PT in the hallway. I stood nearby as they whispered to each other. I saw them nodding their heads and both PTs turned to me. One of them asked me to explain why I couldn't use the assistive devices.

> "By the time I was discharged, I could walk one hundred feet with the use of my walker, before tiring."

I explained that I had to concentrate on maintaining my balance. While standing on one foot, I have to move the other foot and the cane at the same time. There were too many motions, all at the same time. With that, they both turned away while again negatively shaking their heads. At that point, I made statement: "We haven't tried me walking without anything!"

Upon hearing that, they both began shaking their heads. One said, "You can't just go from walking with the assistance of a walker, to walking without anything!" At this time, the other PT spoke up and explained that they were trained to use other assistive devices before letting the patient walk on their own. I asked them to give me a week.

Both PTs remained skeptical of me

ever being able to walk without any assisted devices however, with their expertise and my determination, I went on to walk as I do now. I wholeheartedly credit my ability to walk today to my OT at NER, and the two PTs at Westside, for allowing themselves to think outside of the box, so I can walk as I do now. In August of 2009 I was discharged from Westside.

Since then, my life has pretty much gotten back on track.

Had it not been for rehabilitation after my heart attack and subsequent strokes, I wouldn't be alive today. I know that people who are left in a vegetative state don't live long. Despite many months of hard work, Goodwill also taught me how to go from my disability controlling my life, to me taking control of my disability. Today, my life would never be as productive as it is now, had it not been for the rehabilitative care I received and for that I am truly grateful.

Meet Ralph Poland

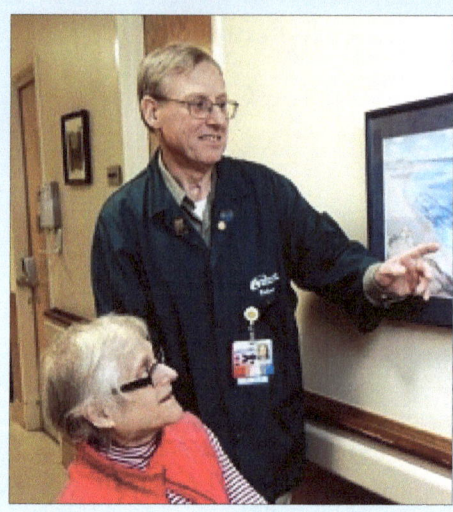

Since re-inventing himself the past seven years, Ralph now works part time at a local Wal-Mart. He also volunteers at a local hospital. His real passion is volunteering at the Rehab where he recovered. There, he shares his story with patients, offering them hope and inspiration.

Ralph also serves on the BIA-MAINE Chapter, as well as on CMMC's Patient Advisory Council. He continues to offer insight from a brain injured survivor's perspective to support groups, Neuro OT students at UNE, and staff members at CMMC.

The TBI HOPE Network continues to evolve and grow, ever mindful of our mission - to Advocate, Educate, and Serve all Affected by Brain Injury.

We are always looking for new and innovative methods to advocate for those who need it most – those impacted by brain injury. Within a few weeks, we expect to launch the new TBI HOPE smartphone app.

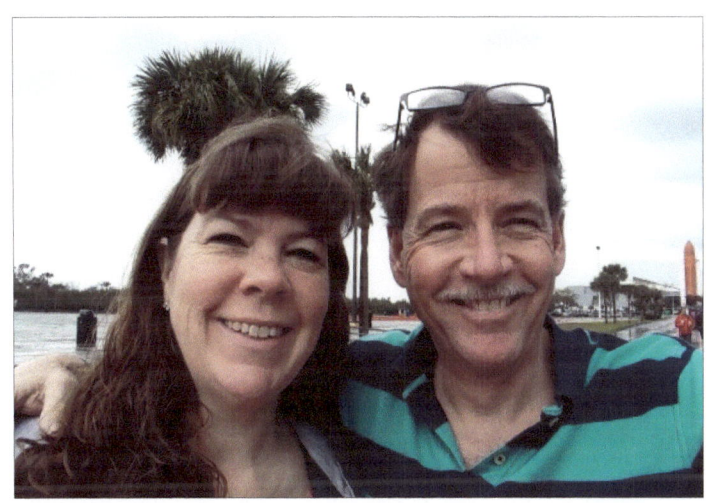

This nifty little app will let users view the current issue of our magazine directly through the app, provide quick access to all past issues as well as more functionality making our content readily available with an easy screen tap.

You've already read that next month, we'll be premiering a printed copy of our magazine to readers. I'll let you in on a little secret. Later this month, we are "soft launching" the print version of TBI HOPE Magazine. Call it a test-run if you will. Expect more information by month end.

Our best wishes for health and happiness to you,

David & Sarah

www.ingramcontent.com/pod-product-compliance
Lightning Source LLC
Chambersburg PA
CBHW041534280526
45792CB00004B/1505